WEIGHT LOSS ESSENTIAL OIL REFERENCE GUIDE

Burn belly fat, lose weight, boost immune system and metabolism with specialized weight loss essential oils.

Jeffery O. Thomsen

WEIGHT LOSS ESSENTIAL OIL REFERENCE GUIDE:

Burn belly fat, lose weight, boost immune system and metabolism with specialized weight loss essential oils.

Jeffery O. Thomsen

Copyright © January 2019

All rights reserved

This book or parts thereof may not be reproduced in any form, stored in a retrieval system, or transmitted in any form by any means: photocopy, electronic, recording, mechanical or otherwise without the written permission of the author.

Contents

Introduction 1

1 Benefits of essential oils 3

2 Understanding carrier oil 10

3 Essential oils for losing weight and various methods of using them 17

4 Essential oil recipes to fasten your weight loss goals (body massages, oil baths, foot scrub, exfoliator, detoxifier, etc.) and improve your general health 49

5 Safety precautions 68

Bonus 1: The Expanded Water Solution Plan (EWSP) for Weight Loss 70

Bonus 2: Daily workout plan to keep fit [a kind reminder!] 74

Conclusion 76

Supporting research 79

Other books by same author ERROR! BOOKMARK NOT DEFINED.

INTRODUCTION

Aromatherapy refers to the act of using scented substances including essential oils for their therapeutic or medicinal benefits. Essential oils are processed extracts from plant's leaves, barks, stalks, rind, flowers, and roots. Since essential oils are highly concentrated and may be harmful if used without diluting them, they are mixed or diluted with carrier oils, such as olive oil, coconut oil, lotion, etc. In application, they can either be applied directly on the skin, through diffusion using an essential oil diffuser, inhaled, or ingested following the US Food and Drug Administration (FDA) recommendations on safety of such essential oil and also taking them as recommended.

Essential oils can be used to treat lots of ailments by following strict recommendations. They can trigger our senses and are beneficial as topical products; they can also repel insects, kill germs, viruses, fungi, and bacteria. Some essential oils are safe to be taken internally according to FDA classification of them. Nevertheless, caution has to be applied when taking essential oils internally especially as pointed out in this book.

If you read this piece to the end, you'll discover additional two more natural yet effective methods you can use to complement your weight loss goals. I added these to make you see the result of your effort within a shorter time. Essential oils have worked for many and you'd never be an exception. Read, apply as recommend and watchout for result.

CHAPTER ONE

BENEFITS OF ESSENTIAL OILS

The many inherent properties of essential oils give rise to many ways they can be used to benefit our health. This book only focuses on a minimal benefit of using essential oils. Remember that the refined drugs we buy from the drug stores are all plant products, but we hardly think in this direction seeing them appear so clean and well packaged. Essential oils are many with many health benefits too. We can't exhaust the benefits of essential oils, but we'll attempt to list just a few. The benefits listed here are for the generality of essential oils and not for some specific ones.

[1] Essential oils are anti-bacterial

Some essential oils have anti-bacterial properties. They can be employed to fight to reduce or remove completely harmful bacteria from the body. Anti-bacterial can destroy a bacterium or inhibit bacteria growth in the body. This can work by preventing them from building a cell wall or merely attacking bacteria cell membranes.

[2] Essential oils are anti-oxidant

Anti-oxidants protect the body against harmful toxins. They get rid of these toxins through perspiration inducement and urination. Anti-oxidants can boost the immune system due to Vitamin C.

[3] Anti-septic nature of essential oil

Essential oil gotten from grapefruit, for example, can be used in cleaning wounds and preventing infection due to its antiseptic property. Anti-septic can also be used in cleaning the home. It can also be used to treat acne or reduce bruises.

[4] Essential oils are antiviral

Antivirals fight to reduce or completely remove viruses from the body especially those present in the mouth, stomach or the digestive system.

[5] Essential oils can be used to tackle depression and anxiety

Essential oils can be used effectively to fight depression and anxiety. Depression and anxiety arise due to extreme emotional changes in our body that goes beyond our control. Essential oils have proved to create calmness, relief stress and uplift our mood and as such can be a perfect solution for depression and anxiety. It can create a positive feeling and relaxes both body and mind.

[6] Essential oils can serve as digestive aids

Essential oils can boost metabolism and help detoxify the digestive system of the body. It can remove bacteria and viruses that are otherwise harmful to the body. It can also deal perfectly well with bloating and cramping.

[7] They can serve as disinfectants

Essential oils can reduce or eliminate from the body or on solid surfaces bacteria and viruses that are harmful and also fight infections.

[8] They can boost energy

Direct inhalation of essential oil can kill tensions caused by certain hormones in the brain and awaken your mental focus to function effectively. It can crash headaches, migraine, mental fatigue, insomnia and depression leading to energy pickup.

[9] Essential oil for hair care

Many essential oils can be used for taking care of the hair. Such care can range from cleaning, growing, killing dandruff beneath it to removing too much oil from it or making it glow. It can also give protection from bacteria for the hair and your head.

[10] Essential oils works excellent for pain and inflammation

Where there are pains and swellings, an essential oil can help bring calm. Through an increased blood flow and circulation, healing cells can quickly be dispatched to where they are needed to make for fast healing of inflamed areas of the body. It can also heal muscle inflammations, PMS cramping or sores.

[11] Essential oils are potent for weight loss

Many essential oils, when used correctly, can suppress appetite, reduce cravings and curb late-night food. They can also boost digestion, burn fat or help the body to produce only fat that can burn on their own. Essential oils can also work great for blood glucose cellulite reduction.

[12] They are perfect for skin care

A single or combination of essential oils can see your skin glowing through natural cleaning due to consistent use and removing dead skin cells. It can also shield it from harmful toxins and ultraviolet rays' damage.

CHAPTER TWO

UNDERSTANDING CARRIER OIL

Carrier oils are vegetable oils derived from plant's fatty parts. These parts are usually its seeds, nuts or kernels. Freshly extracted essential oils are undiluted and highly concentrated capable of reacting adversely or causing irritation if used topically or taken internally. As a result, they must be diluted before applying on skin. This is where the concept of carrier oil comes in. Hence, carrier oils are used to reduce the effect of the highly concentrated essential oils. Depending on what you want to achieve with essential oils, different carrier oils can be recommended.

Carrier oils are not used only with essentials oils; creams, body lotions, bath and body oils, balms, etc. are also carried with carrier oils. Since the ability of essential oils to work effectively depends to a large extent on the nature of carrier oil used for dilution, the discussion here is of utmost importance.

Carrier oils can play a big part in the result or effect of our essential oils. It can make a difference in the aroma, color, therapeutic properties or shelf life of your finished product. It is vital that we pay attention to how to use carrier oils with our essential oils to achieve the maximum result. Take note that "carrier oils" as a name are only used in the practice of aromatherapy. Outside of aromatherapy, these oils are referred to as a vegetable, base or fixed oils. However, vegetable oils are only from vegetarian sources whereas base and fixed oils are not and are mostly not used in aromatherapy.

The most preferred or best carrier oils for aromatherapy purpose are usually odorless or with a little smell of sweetness; strong or bitter smell point to the fact that they have gone rancid and hence unfit for aromatherapy practice or purpose. Rancidity occurs due to natural fatty acids present in the oil called tocopherols. Method of production can also contribute to the oil becoming rancid. One way to know if carrier oil has become stale is to smell the aroma when you just buy it and compared the smell when you want to use it. Most times, they smell strong and bitter when they have gone rancid. There are many types of carrier oils such as coconut oil, sweet almond oil, moringa oil, jojoba oil, apricot oil, borage seed oil, olive oil, etc. Some of these oils can be picked from grocery stores, but the problem here is that they may not be cold-pressed. Most likely, they are processed with heat and as a result not fit for aromatherapy practice. The best place to get a nourishing and freshest carrier [and essential] oils are specialty stores for aromatherapy ingredients. Buying from health stores can be a little expensive. Ensure you check very well the expiry date during buying and before use. Also, ensure there are no additives blended in. You don't necessarily need to buy carrier oils already mixed with essential oil(s).

Buy only "Cold expeller pressed" or simply "Cold pressed" carrier oils. These measures are to avoid that they were not exposed to much heat. Heat damages the fragile nutrients in carrier oils. If you can, avoid carrier oils labels with "Expeller pressed." It's crucial to have the therapeutic properties of carrier oils when using for aromatherapy purpose. You also need to check how it was extracted. It has to be organically produced and of high quality. Take particular note of the aroma of your carrier oil as it can affect the final scent when blended with essential oils. You don't necessarily need to buy much of carrier oil as they may become rancid with time due to oxidation. Just estimate the quantity you need at any particular time and use all at once. Be careful and refused to be convinced to go for mineral oils. Mineral oils aren't natural, and their process of extraction doesn't qualify them for aromatherapy purpose. They can easily clog the skin pores preventing it from breathing from the essential oil applied to it. Once the skin is prevented from breathing naturally, it becomes difficult for it to excrete toxins through sweating.

Storage of carrier oils should be kept away from sunlight. Store in a cool and dark place and also in a dark airtight fitting glass bottle, e.g., cobalt Boston. Please take note that storage in dark bottles is meant for prolong period [even though not recommended]. If you plan to use them within a short period, this may not be necessary. The manufacturer may send them to you in plastic containers for economic reasons. Don't see it as being of low quality. On the other hand, essential oils should also be kept in glass bottles and NOT plastic. It can dissolve or pick up the scent of the plastic container rendering it useless for aromatherapy. Storage of carrier oils in a refrigerator is recommended. If it solidifies inside the fridge, leave it outside to have it return to normal before use.

CHAPTER THREE

ESSENTIAL OILS FOR LOSING WEIGHT AND VARIOUS METHODS OF USING THEM

[1.] GRAPEFRUIT ESSENTIAL OIL

Research conducted by Shen J. et al. (2005) suggests that grapefruit can help suppress appetite and hence reduce body weight. The grapefruit essential oil is gotten from the rind or fresh peel of the grapefruit. It is an appetite suppressant, fat dissolver, a detoxifier and can also prevent body water retention and bloating. The rind of grapefruit contains nootkatone in high concentration – a constituent that activates AMPK (Murase T. et al. (2010). This substance arouses the body system to consume more sugar and also reduces fat accumulation. The whole process works to reduce body weight. As more fat keeps burning and more sugar used up, weight loss becomes a natural reality. Grapefruit essential oil when used effectively also support metabolism, reduce desire for food and burns body fat. The FDA approves it for internal use.

Application

Method 1: Taken internally

Pure grapefruit oil is mixed with water and taken on the go. Recommended quantity is one drop to a glassful of water. This should be taken 15-20 minutes before a meal to improve digestion, burn out fat and reduce cravings for food. Take note that oil generally can't mix with water by putting them together. Hence, to cross the hurdle, take one teaspoon or a tablespoon of aloe vera gel and dissolve the oil in it. Mix thoroughly with the aloe-vera gel before adding a recommended quantity of water. That's just one way to mix an essential oil with water. You can also use aloe vera juice if the gel isn't readily available.

Method 2: Direct inhalation

You can inhale the aroma of grapefruit essential oil to kill sudden cravings. Inhalation can be done directly from the oil bottle or adding a few drops to a cotton ball or handkerchief and breathing in deeply from it.

The smell relaxes the body's mechanism of activating food cravings or sending hunger signals from the parasympathetic gastric nerve.

Method 3: Topical application

The grapefruit oil can also be rubbed on the wrist, temples, chest, and beneath the nose. This can help control your cravings and suppress your appetite.

Method 4: Using a diffuser

To your diffusing device, add 2-3 drops of the grapefruit oil and let it diffuse out and fill the atmosphere of your room. This can greatly restrain late-night cravings which aren't recommended as a general feeding rule.

[2.] THE CINNAMON ESSENTIAL OIL

A study conducted by Ranasinghe P. et al. (2013) posited that Cinnamon "has anti-parasitic, anti-oxidant, anti-microbial, and free radical scavenging properties." They suggested that it can "reduce blood glucose and serum cholesterol." Nitsa Mirsky (2012) also suggests that the Cinnamon oil can regulate blood glucose levels and glucose tolerance factor (GTF) in the human body. It's a fact that unbalanced blood glucose or sugar levels can cause over-eating, cravings for sugar, energy level drop, weight gain and even irritability. Few drops of Cinnamon essential oil to a portion of food can slow down the speed at which glucose get into the bloodstream and consequently assisting the body to gain less weight in the long run.

Research by Sigh et al. (2007) also shows that the oil from Cinnamon leaf contains Eugenol. Eugenol is a component that can act on the body's neurosensory perceptions and alter our sense of smell and taste towards food which subsequently suppresses cravings and over-eating. Cinnamon is anti-oxidant, anti-diabetic, anti-inflammatory, anti-microbial, lipid-lowering, anti-cancer, etc. For this work, we'll focus on its application for losing weight. When it comes to cravings suppression, Cinnamon has it. Subsequent works can cover how Cinnamon can be used for other health challenges.

Application

Method 1: Taken internally

The US Food and Drug Administration (FDA) classifies Cinnamon essential oil safe to be taken internally. In addition to this classification, such Cinnamon oil must be hundred percent pure, toxin- and additive-free, undiluted and unfiltered. This rule applies to all essential oils that are recommended by the FDA to be taken internally. To burn fat, get raw honey (just a pint of it) and add into a teacup filled with warm water. Add 1-2 drops of Cinnamon essential oil to it. Stir it and drink while still warm. Take these 10-20 minutes before a meal to reduce cravings. You can also take it at night to check cravings. If possible, add to your oats or smoothies. To dissolve your oil in water, take a pinch of sea salt and add the recommended drops of your essential oil to it. Mix them thoroughly together before adding water so that the oil mixes completely.

Method 2: Direct inhalation

You can condition your system to eat little and still be satisfied. To kill sudden food cravings or prevent or prevent overeating, breathe intensely right from the bottle of Cinnamon essential oil. This works best to curb emotional eating habit and can also go a long way to improve your mood.

Method 3: Topical application

To use Cinnamon essential oil typically, you must combine it with a carrier oil. You can go for olive or coconut oil as a carrier. Add 1-2 drops of Cinnamon essential oil to the carrier oil of your choice. Stir and allow it to sit for 5-10 minutes. Rub and massage it on your chest and wrists.

Method 4: Using a diffuser

To your diffuser bottle, add 2-3 drops of Cinnamon essential oil and make the aroma fill your space. The scent is great. This can curb night cravings. As you continue, your passion for a night or midnight food would drastically reduce and possibly cease. One primary reason why night carving is frown at is that of the body's inability to digest what's taken properly before morning. This is a dangerous eating habit that's responsible for most people's weight gain. When you don't eat right, the food becomes a burden for the body.

[3.] GINGER ESSENTIAL OIL

Ginger is anti-inflammatory. Reduced inflammations result to better digestion and absorption of nutrients in the body. This is especially important if weight loss is to be achieved. Gingerols, a compound in ginger reduces inflammations and leads to better absorption. As a result, diseases are prevented. Most times, disease sets in due to undigested food particles in the body. Losing weight requires general good health. Ginger possesses anti-oxidant, anti-inflammatory and antinociceptive properties. This was confirmed by Jeena K. et al. (2013) in a study. Again, a study conducted by Saravanan G. et al. (2014) suggests that the presence of gingerol is effective for curing obesity. Indeed, ginger essential oil can help with weight loss.

Application
Method 1: Taken internally

Again, the FDA classifies ginger essential oil safe for internal use. However, as I said earlier, it must be hundred percent pure and preferably used with warm water. To a glass of it, add 1-2 drops of ginger essential oil. Add little raw honey and a fresh juice of lemon fruit. Drink it before meal time. Again, you can use a pinch of baking soda as a dispersant for your oil before adding water. Go ahead; you have three choices now to use and mix your essential oil with water. Choose whichever you love.

Method 2: Direct inhalation

To curb cravings and keep your appetite in check, breathe directly from the ginger essential oil bottle.

[4.] PEPPERMINT ESSENTIAL OIL

The peppermint oil is one of the most common essential oil. It is most commonly used in treating indigestion. When combined with caraway oil, it can relax the stomach muscles and also decrease bloating (Goerg KJ et al., 2003). Menthol, the cooling compound in peppermint is perfect for digestion and calming an upset stomach. Most importantly, menthol can affect the neuro-sensors to change our sense of taste and smell of food, preventing cravings and also curbing over-eating. Research has shown that peppermint scent can significantly suppress food cravings. Peppermint is not recommended for topical application especially around the eyes.

Application
Method 1: Taken internally

The FDA also classifies peppermint oil to be safe for taking it internally. Add 1-2 drops of peppermint oil to a glassful of water. This should be taken before 15-20 minutes before mealtime to suppress your appetite. Remember, to go for a hundred percent pure peppermint oil which should be free of additives and toxins; they are also undiluted and unfiltered. Disperse your essential oil in 1 tablespoon of aloe-vera gel before adding water to it. Make sure you mix the two things thoroughly.

Method 2: Direct inhalation

Inhale directly and deeply from the peppermint essential oil bottle. This can significantly suppress your food cravings leading to weight loss. This has to be done 15-20 before meal time.

Method 3: Using a diffuser

Add 3-4 drops of peppermint essential oil to a diffuser and make the aroma fill the space of your room. You'll especially love the minty scent.

[5.] LEMON ESSENTIAL OIL

The lemon essential oil is extracted from the rind of a lemon fruit. It works great with the immune, digestive and respiratory systems.

When combined with grapefruit essential oil, lemon oil can be used to suppress body weight gain (Akira N. et al., 2003).

Application

Method 1: Taken internally

Lemon essential oil can be ingested according to FDA classification. Add 1-2 drops to a glass of warm water and take it early in the morning to aid digestion. Lemon essential oil is especially effective for detoxification as well. Follow any of the methods above to dissolve your essential oil in water.

Method 2: Direct inhalation

To curb cravings and keep your appetite in check, breathe directly from the lemon essential oil bottle. You can as well take few drops and have it a cotton ball then inhale from there.

Method 3: Body Massage

Mix lemon essential oil (2-3 drops) with a carrier oil such as olive or coconut oil. Rub and massage your body with it to cause the skin to breathe and firm up.

[6.] BERGAMOT ESSENTIAL OIL

The Bergamot essential oil can be used to fight anxiety and depressive feelings. It acts by reducing cortisol to bring about positive mood (Watanabe E. et al., 2015). It's a fact that anxiety and depressive can contribute significantly to emotional eating to satisfy your feeling which then results in weight gain. A study conducted by Mollace V. et al. (2011) suggested that Bergamot can reduce blood cholesterol and blood glucose significantly. Bergamot essential oil can melt fat as well as sugar in the body through a compound called polyphenols which is highly effective for losing weight. Bergamot also has limonene concentrations in large quantity which can help dissolve fat preventing weight gain.

Application
Method 1: Direct inhalation

Inhale the Bergamot essential oil deeply directly or through a cotton ball with 2-3 drops of Bergamot oil soaked with it. The scent is a powerful appetite suppressant.

Method 2: Using a diffuser

Add 1-2 drops of Bergamot oil to your diffuser and let the aroma fill the space of your room. The citrus scent can relax the nerves, uplift mood and suppress cravings.

Method 3: Body bath

Add 3-4 drops of Bergamot essential oil to your shower and get soaked and inhale deeply from it.

[7.] SANDALWOOD ESSENTIAL OIL

Sandalwood essential oil works best for emotional eaters that may be suffering from anxiety and depression. Most times, anxiety and depression are due to hormonal changes. Fortunately, the Sandalwood essential oil has a therapeutic effect that works to balance hormones in the brain that unduly triggers hunger due to emotions. Sandalwood essential oil can be inhaled directly, applied topically or added to a diffuser.

Application

Method 1: Direct inhalation

Sandalwood has an earthy scent which can cause instant relaxation of the body system and keep you in peace. Direct inhalation from the bottle is recommended to curb cravings.

Method 2: Topical application

Rub and massage your wrist, chest, and muscles to reduce cravings.

Method 3: Using a diffuser

Add 1-2 drops to your diffuser to calm your nerves and reduce your cravings after a long day.

[8.] LEVANDER ESSENTIAL OIL

Are you addicted to binge or emotional eating? Lavender oil can be of great help. Lavender oil can relax the nerves and inhibit a feeling of anxiety and depression. Lavender essential oil is mostly applied through direct inhalation, body massage as they are quickly absorbed from the skin (Jager et al., 2002) or using essential oil diffuser. Research shows that Lavender essential oil possesses anti-depressive, anticonvulsant, sedative, anxiolytic and calming properties (Cavanagh H.M.A. et al., 2002; Gorji A. et al., 2001; Gorji A., 2003).

Application

Method 1: Direct inhalation

Take a few drops (1-2) of Lavender oil and soak it in a cotton ball for breath or breathe profoundly and directly from the bottle.

Method 2: Using a diffuser

Like other essential oils, add 2-3 drops of Lavender essential oil to your diffuser bottle and let the aroma fills your entire room.

Continuous inhalation calms and relaxes the nerves and reduces food cravings.

[9.] FENNEL ESSENTIAL OIL

Fennel essential oil has a sweet, earthy smell. The oil is gotten from the Fennel seed through distillation. Fennel oil is especially great for suppressing appetite, regulating sleep cycle and improving digestion. Fennel oil contains melatonin hormone which regulates circulation rhythms and also triggers the brain sleep cycles. A study conducted by Agil A. et al. (2011) suggest that melatonin can trigger the body to produce fat that can only burn and not get stored leading to weight gain. Fennel oil is also found to speed up digestion. Two methods exist for application of Fennel essential oil to lose weight.

Application

Method 1: Taken internally

Within 15-20 minutes just before a meal, take a glass of water mixed with 1-2 drops of Fennel essential oil and drink it to prevent over-eating and improve digestion. Follow recommended method to disperse oil in water before drinking.

Method 2: Topical application

Dab, rub and massage Fennel oil on both wrists and temples to curb cravings.

[10.] EUCALYPTUS ESSENTIAL OIL

Eucalyptus oil can reduce stress, boost energy and invigorate the senses. It has a refreshing minty aroma and can reduce mental fatigue. It directly alleviates anxiety and stress which positively impact on over-eating and weight gain. The scent of eucalyptus lessens urge for food and also kill stress feelings.

Application

Method 1: Direct inhalation

You can directly inhale it from the bottle or soak few drops with a cotton ball. The immediate result is calmness and relaxation in your body and brain preventing you from emotional eating.

Method 2: Body bath

Add 2-3 drops of eucalyptus oil to your shower. Cover the drain and breathe in deeply to get refreshed and become mentally sound.

BY THE WAY, don't get scared that the whole idea of using essential oils to fight weight gain is targeted at fighting cravings and reducing food intake. The fact is that our body doesn't want that it be overloaded with food. Just a little food at the right time is enough to keep you going. What you need is a water intake plan to detoxify and keeps your system clean always. A proper water intake plan can help you lose weight considerably and keep you in good health all year long. But the problem is that most people don't get to like it. Hence, using essential oils to suppress cravings is indeed a good idea to lose weight and perfect when combined with a water intake plan.

[11.] FRANKINCENSE ESSENTIAL OIL

This oil is excellent for keeping your anxiousness in check that could otherwise trigger cravings. Frankincense oil can as well speed up digestion and help you lose weight.

Application
Method 1: Direct inhalation

To kill cravings for food or emotional eating, breathe deeply and directly from the oil bottle. You can also soak few drops with a cotton ball and breathe from there.

Method 2: Using a diffuser

Fill your room space with the sweet aroma of Frankincense oil. Just add 2-3 drops of it to your diffuser bottle. This is especially beautiful to be used after a long working day to reduce stress and cravings for food.

[12.] JASMINE ESSENTIAL OIL

The Jasmine oil is gotten from the Jasmine flower. It has a calming smell. Jasmine can be great for uplifting mood, relieving depression (Hongratanaworakit, 2010). It can also help with insomnia. Once anxiety and depression can be controlled, it becomes easy to lose weight.

Application

Method 1: Direct inhalation

Direct inhalation before a meal can create calmness and curb over-eating. You can also make 2-3 drops into your handkerchief and use it on the go.

Method 2: Using a diffuser

Jasmine is also perfect to be used through a diffuser. You can equally combine it with grapefruit oil. Introduce 2-3 and 4-5 drops of Jasmine and grapefruit oil respectively into your diffuser. The scent coming out from the diffuser would be so satisfying and have the parasympathetic gastric nerve relaxed. This nerve usually creates food cravings and needs to be put in check. The aroma coming out of the diffuser is also mood uplifting.

[12.] ORANGE ESSENTIAL OIL

A study carried out in Japan's Mei University proves orange oil to lessen anti-depressant medication intake. Orange has anti-oxidant properties and can prevent cravings for food. It's a fact that depression is directly proportional to weight gain and if orange can work positively to reduce anti-depressant medication; then it can be a good choice for weight loss.

Application

Method 1: Taken internally

Orange essential oil has the backing of the FDA to be taken internally. Following any recommended ways of mixing oil with water, introduce 1-2 drops of orange essential oil to a glassful of water and take immediately before mealtime to keep your appetite in check and prevent over-eating by creating a sense of satisfaction with a little food that you eat.

Method 2: Direct inhalation

Breathe deeply and directly from the orange essential oil bottle minutes before food to stimulate your senses and to prevent over-eating.

[14.] ROSEMARY ESSENTIAL OIL

Rosemary essential oil can decrease stress hormones (cortisol). This discovery was made from a study carried out in Atsumi T. et al. (2007). The study posits that high cortisol level is directly proportional to high-stress levels that can result in mindless eating.

Application

Method 1: Direct inhalation

Direct inhalation from the bottle should be carried out to decrease cortisol levels leading to drop in stress levels. This should be done up to 5 times at a go.

Method 2: Using a diffuser

You can also make 2-3 drops of Rosemary essential oil into your diffuser and make the aroma fill up your room to relief you from stress and curb your cravings.

CHAPTER FOUR

ESSENTIAL OIL RECIPES TO FASTEN YOUR WEIGHT LOSS GOALS (BODY MASSAGES, OIL BATHS, FOOT SCRUB, ETC.) AND IMPROVE YOUR GENERAL HEALTH

1. Anti-cellulite cream:

The grapefruit essential oil is effective for preventing water retention in the body and stimulate a system that transport fluid or water towards the heart (lymphatic system). Grapefruit also contain the bromelin (anti-inflammatory) enzyme that can help in breaking down cellulite. This is the major reason this fruit is used in cellulite creams. You can easily prepare a cellulite cream using grapefruit essential oil at home.

Requirements:

- **Thirty** drops of grapefruit essential oil
- **One** cup of olive oil
- **A** glass jar

Instructions for preparation and use:

- Add together the two ingredients in a glass jar and mix them thoroughly.
- Allow the mixture to sit for **thirty** minutes.
- Rub and massage directly on the areas of your body with cellulite (dimpled flesh on thighs, buttocks, hips and stomach) that needs to be firmed for **five** minutes daily.

2. Preparing a grapefruit sugar scrub

Sugar scrubs moisturizes and exfoliates the skin making it silky. It can be used on the whole body to open up skin pores which is necessary so that the skin can breathe in the essential oils through baths, massage or diffusion.

Requirements:

- **Half** cup of granulated sugar (organic sugar preferably).
- **Half** cup of olive or coconut oil.
- **Ten** drops of grapefruit essential oil.
- **A** glass jar.

Instructions for preparation and use:

- Add together all the ingredients above in a glass jar and mix thoroughly.
- Use the preparation as you may wish in the shower.
- Store in an airtight glass jar.

3. Grapefruit oil body wash

Requirements:

- **Sixty** drops of grapefruit essential oil.
- **One** cup of liquid castile soap.

- **One-fourth** cup of raw honey.
- **Two** teaspoonful of olive oil.
- **One** teaspoonful of Vitamin E. oil
- Squirt container bottle.

Instructions for preparation and use:

- Add together all the ingredients above in a glass jar and mix thoroughly.

- Turn everything into a squirt bottle and make to sit for **thirty** minutes.

- Shake before every use.

- Squirt or drop the preparation onto a bath pouf, washed cloth or directly on skin and rub gently.

4. Skin tightening lotion

This also works great to break down cellulite and firm up your skin.

Requirements:

- **Twelve** ounces (oz) natural lotion (unscented), e.g., shea butter lotion.

- **Twenty** drops of grapefruit essential oil.
- **Fifteen** drops of peppermint essential oil.
- **Fifteen** drops of lime essential oil.
- **A** glass jar.

Instructions for preparation and use:

- Fill **six** ounces (oz) shea butter lotion in a glass jar.
- Add the grapefruit essential oil into it and mix thoroughly.
- Add the peppermint essential oil and continue mixing.
- Do same for lime essential oil.
- Add the remaining **six** ounces shea butter lotion and stir thoroughly.
- Use as needed.

5. DIY lavender soap bars

Lavender is known to arrest anxiety and curb emotional eating in the process. Using it as a bathing soap can be extremely supporting to other methods.

Requirements:

- **Thirty** drops of lavender essential oil.
- Soap base, e.g., goat's milk.
- **Three** drops of Vitamin E oil.
- Soap mold.

Instructions for preparation and use:

- Set a medium heat and place a pot of water on it.
- Put the soap base inside a container and place it just above the water inside the pot and give minutes to melt.
- Bring down the melted soap base and allow it to cool.
- Introduce the lavender and vitamin E oil to it and mix it thoroughly.
- Pour into soap molds.
- Allow to cool then bring them out from the molds.

- It's ready for use.
- Store at room temperature.

6. DIY rash cream

Requirements:

- **One-fourth** cup of cocoa butter.
- **One-eight** cup of grapeseed oil.
- **Two** tablespoonful of bentonite clay.
- **Two** tablespoonful aloevera gel.
- **Ten** drops of lavender essential oil.
- **Two** tablespoonful of witch hazel.

Instruction for preparation and use:

- On a low heat, melt both the cocoa butter oil with the grape seed oil. Stir thoroughly to mix well.

- Introduce the aloevera gel and stir well.
- Get it off the heat, introduce the bentonite clay, witch hazel and lavender essential oil and mix well.

- Transfer into container with cover and close.
- Make it sit for **thirty** minutes.
- Rub on the affected area with it.
- Leave for **fifteen-twenty** minutes on skin.
- Dab small towel or handkerchief into warm water and clean the area.

<u>Caution:</u> Known allergic to mint herbs should apply caution in use of this preparation.

7. DIY headache inhaler

To get relief from headache, why not prepare an inhaler from combination of essential oils? This is purely natural and works great to tune the senses.

Requirements:

- **Two** drops of frankincense essential oil.
- **Seven** drops of lavender essential oil.

- **Three** drops of ravintsara essential oil.
- **Three** drops of fir essential oil.
- Inhaler stick.

Instructions for preparation and use:

- Get a little container and add all the ingredients into it.
- Mix thoroughly and pour it into your inhaler stick.
- Use as needed when headache strikes.

8. Weight loss capsule

Just by taking this capsule, you will begin to see a drop in your weight within a month. Purely natural yet works! Listen to your body and discontinue immediately if you notice adverse effect.

Requirements:

- **Two** drops of lemon essential oil.
- **Two** drops of grapefruit essential oil.

- **Two** drops of peppermint essential oil.
- **Twelve** drops of liquid fractionated coconut oil.
- Empty gel capsules.
- An eye dropper.

Instructions for preparation and use:

- Put together the essentials along with the liquid fractionated coconut oil in a glass container and mix thoroughly.
- Use an eye dropper to add the mixture to the gel capsules.
- Take **one** capsule **twenty** minutes before breakfast. Three days a week (one or two days in-between).
- You can multiply ingredients for more capsules to cover more days.

9. Combination diffuser blend to curb appetite

Requirements:

- **Three** drops of grapefruit essential oil.

- **Three** drops of lemon essential oil.
- **One** drop of spear mint essential oil.
- **One** drop of rose essential oil.

Instruction for preparation and use:

- Mix all the essential oils listed above and pour into a diffuser.
- Diffuse **one to two** hours before meal to reduce cravings and prevent over-eating.

10.   Weight loss foot rub

Requirements:

- **Four** drops of lavender oil.
- **Ten** drops of grapefruit essential oil.
- **Three** drops of juniper essential oil.
- **Four** drops of basil essential oil.
- **Five** drops of cypress essential oil.
- **Two** teaspoonful of olive or coconut oil.
- A beaker or small glass bottle.

Instruction for preparation and use:

- Put together the listed ingredients in a beaker or small glass bottle.
- Rub and massage on your feet every night before sleep.
- You can also add to bath water.
- Multiplied ingredients for more use.

11. Weight loss massage oil

Requirements:

- **Forty** drops of grapefruit essential oil.
- **Thirty** drops of lemon essential oil.
- **Thirty** drops of geranium essential oil.
- **Thirty** drops of rose essential oil.
- **One** ounce liquid fractionated coconut oil.
- **A** squirt bottle.

Instruction for preparation and use:

- Put together all the ingredients listed above in a squirt bottle and mix thoroughly.

- Allow to sit for **thirty** minutes.
- Use as a body massage oil.

12. Tummy tuck cream

Requirements:

- **Fifteen** drops of lavender, grapefruit, geranium, and frankincense essential oils.
- **One** cup of olive oil.
- **One-eight** cup of vitamin E oil.
- **One-fourth** cup of grated beeswax.
- **One** cup of rose water.

Instructions for preparation and use:

- Using a double boiler, pour the ingredients into a clean pot and place on it with exception of rose water and essentials oils.

- Allow the mixture to melt over a medium heat.

- Turn the mixture into a blender and let it cool at room temperature before blending it.

- Blend it until it mixes thoroughly after cooling.
- Make sure to scrape in the sides as you do.
- Add the rose water and keep blending to have it thoroughly mixed.
- Introduce the essential oils and keep blending.
- Turn the cream into airtight container(s).
- Rub and massage over belly to tighten and reduce fat.

13. DIY exfoliating foot scrub

Foot scrubs are used to exfoliate the foot and remove dead skin. The mixture used here is perfect for what it does. Olive oil possesses anti-inflammatory and anti-oxidant properties while Vitamin E is a moisturizing agent; coconut oil is anti-microbial whereas tea tree is great for healing the skin. Peppermint and lavender can help with great sense of relaxation on your foot relieving aches and pains. Instead of buying this costly in the marketplace, you can easily prepare a foot scrub at home.

Requirements:

- **One and a half** cup of sea salt.
- **One** tablespoon of olive oil.
- **Two** tablespoon of coconut oil.
- **Five** drops of tea tree essential oil.
- **Five** drops of peppermint essential oil.
- **Eight** drops of lavender essential oil.
- **A** glass jar.

Instruction for preparation and use:

- Using a bowl, add and mix the coconut and olive oils.
- Introduce the essential oils and mix well.

- Transfer your mixture into a glass jar and close it tightly to prevent air from entering.

- Keep away from children in a cool dark place.

- Take over **twenty-four** ounces for each use.

- Use as foot scrub for over **fifteen** minutes in the shower before rinsing off with warm water.

- Allow your foot to dry on its own.

14. Preparing a bubble bath

Research suggests that blood sugar can be regulated by simply submerging the body to heat. Bubble bath relaxes greatly and improve mood. It also ensures the best of the therapeutic properties of essential oils get into our system to produce required effects.

Requirements:

- **Half** cup light almond oil.
- **One** egg white.
- **One-fourth** cup of honey.
- **Half** cup of liquid castile soap.
- **Half** teaspoon chamomile essential oil.
- **Half** teaspoon lavender essential oil.

Instruction for preparation and use:

- Using a glass jar, add the egg, almond oil and honey and mix thoroughly.

- Add the essential and Castile soap.

- Mix everything thoroughly [using a spoon or fork].

- Store in a refrigerator.

- Take over **twenty-six** ounces per bath.

15.   Preparing a grapefruit juice

Grapefruit juice is nutritious and refreshing and very effective with weight loss. Grapefruit contains no cholesterol, no sodium, has low calories, loaded with Vitamin A and C and rich in lycopene which is an antioxidant. Grapefruit can help greatly for detoxification and weight loss.

Requirements:
- **Two or three** pieces of grapefruit.
- **A** juicer.
- **One** tablespoonful of honey.

Instruction for preparation and use:
- Rinse them in warm water.
- Cut each one into half.
- Place each half in a juicer.
- Pour the juice into a pitcher.
- Add honey to reduce bitterness (optional).
- Cover the pitcher and store in a fridge to chill.
- Consume as desire.

16. Lavender body massage oil

Lavender is highly tolerable and safe (Perry R. et al, 2012; Dwyer, A.V. et al, 2011) and can be used in a variety of ways including massage to curb binge or emotional eating. It also works great to curb insomnia (Hirokawa, K. et al, 2012).

Requirements:
- **Forty** drops of lavender essential oil.
- **One** ounce liquid fractionated coconut oil.
- **A** squirt bottle.

Instruction for preparation and use:
- Put together all the ingredients listed above in a squirt bottle and mix thoroughly.
- Allow to sit for **thirty** minutes.
- Use as a body massage oil.

CHAPTER FIVE

SAFETY PRECAUTIONS

Essential oils are highly potent and can cause adverse effects if used without observing necessary precautions. Always, be careful and guided using essential oils by following the precautions:

1. A patch test should be done by applying essential oil to the leg, arm or behind the ear region to test for irritation or other harmful effects before full usage. Don't simply jump into using them. They can hurt.

2. Pregnant or nursing women should talk to their doctor before using essential oil especially if they will have to use them internally.

3. Always go for hundred percent pure essential oils without addictive.

4. Essential oils are naturally concentrated, dilute or use by instruction. Most recommended for dilution are carrier oils e.g. coconut oil, olive oil, etc.

5. Essential oils such as bergamot, bitter orange, lemon, etc. are photo-sensitive. Avoid them before much exposure to sun. Also, citrus oils, cinnamon bark, etc. can become irritating to skin if used multiple times or if they are not well diluted before used.

6. Essentials oils are flammable. Don't place essential oil bottle near naked flame or fire.

BONUS 1:

CATALYZING YOUR WEIGHT LOSS, FAT BURN AND METABOLISM GOALS WITH EXPANDED WATER SOLUTION PLAN ON (EWSP) WEIGHT LOSS

Water is powerful and can form part of your consideration to lose weight. If you follow all directives dutifully, you will begin to see tangible results on your body and improvement in your overall health as soon as possible. One thing about the EWSP is that it generally works to usher you into a drug-free life; staying in complete natural health.

Most people drink water to quench thirst. On the contrary, drinking water for weight loss is completely different from taking water to quench thirst. Here, water is taken as medicine to heal your body and not just for drinking sake. Don't underestimate the power of drinking water to crash weight, burn fat, detoxify and keep you in complete health.

Now we already know what grapefruit essential oil can do for us regarding weight loss. It's no more news that grapefruit oil tops other essential oils when it comes to weight loss. Aloe-vera, on the other hand, works great as a digestive stimulant. So this method is sure going to get you there, but it's usually tough to follow it up. You will surely need some level of discipline to get this work for you because this is going to be a daily routine.

Requirements:

- **300cl** or 100 ounces water bottle [for the day].

- **A** 150cl or 50 ounces water bottle.

- **A** 75cl or 25 ounces water bottle.

- **Two** drops of grapefruit essential oil.

- **One** tablespoon of aloe vera gel.

Method:

- Get a little cup, add your aloe vera gel into it and disperse your grapefruit essential oil in it. Mix thoroughly to make sure the essential oil completely mix with it before adding water. Add a little water to it, stir and turn everything it into your 300cl or 100 ounce water bottle. Pour in water and fill up the container completely.

- Now fill up your 150cl water bottle. Shake thoroughly and drink everything within **one to three** minutes. You can drink from the water bottle or use a big glass. The time for this should be around 4:00am in the morning.

- Repeat for a 75cl water bottle. The time for this should be around 5:00am in the morning. That's an hour apart. Store the remaining water in a refrigerator for evening.

- Repeat again for a 75cl water bottle in the evening. The time for this should be around 5:00pm. Water should be at room temperature before drinking it.

BONUS 2:

DAILY WORKOUT PLAN TO KEEP FIT [A KIND REMINDER!]

I only want to remind you about this. Daily exercise is indeed good. Don't ignore it. Whatever you do, a workout plan should be part of your daily routine. I highly recommend it as a complement to using essential oils to get some pounds off your body. It shouldn't cost you much; thirty minutes to an hour should just be fine for it. You can do that right? Everybody needs a workout no matter how short the time may be. Don't underestimate the effect an exercise can have on your health. Workout among other things would make you smart and full of energy and stamina. Even if it's a dance around your room enough to make you sweat out is fine. It helps the skin to excrete toxins and breathe freely. Workouts can also help you have a clear mind and works great for your joints and muscles. You don't necessarily need a gym but to shake up your body in such a way to make you sweat and relax your mind and also make your blood circulate as easy as possible.

CONCLUSION

Getting anything done requires determination and consistency. Once those two are in place, the work becomes guaranteed to arrive at an expected end. Now, you don't have to buy and use all the essential oils mention in this book but to read up carefully then choose and stick to one or combine with another that does a different thing to get you to your goals. That would form a plan for you. For instance, if there is no mention of body bath for particular oil and you wish to include a body bath in your program, you can use another essential oil solely for body bath to combine with your main oil(s) or plan that does most of the other things. Trying to buy all the oils can be pocket draining.

Draw up a plan based on what you have read and stick to that considering how much you'll have to spend on a monthly basis to get to your goal. Make your plan concrete and stick to it. Whatever you choose to include in it, I will strongly recommend you add both or at least one of EWSP or workout for a faster result and general good health and fitness. I can't personally come up with a plan for you since our body systems differ. What may work for me may not work for you. Personally

- I diffuse most of the time but not all night. Most times, just for 3 hours and it shuts off automatically, and it's only in my bedroom and not to use and entertain visitors in the sitting room.

- I ingest just three times a week.

- I love the grapefruit juice and I take it often.
- I exfoliate once a month.

- I do body massage two to three times a week.

- The EWSP has always been my daily routine. Sometimes, without the essential oil.

- Lastly, I do cycle or do some workouts early in the morning.

So that's my plan and it has been working great for me. If you love it, you can adopt or draw up one for yourself.

SUPPORTING RESEARCH

Agil A., Navarro-Alarcón M., Ruiz R., Abuhamadah S., El-Mir M.Y., Vázquez G.F. Beneficial effects of melatonin on obesity and lipid profile in young Zucker diabetic fatty rats. J Pineal Res. 2011 Mar; 50(2): 207-12. Doi:10.1111/j.1600-079X.2010.00830.x. Epub 2010 Nov 19.

Akira N., Katsuya N. Effect of olfactory stimulation with flavor of grapefruit oil and lemon oil on the activity of sympathetic branch in the white adipose tissue of the epididymis. SAGE Journals. Available at: http://journals.sagepub.com/doi/abs/10.1177/153537020322801014. First published 1 November 2003.

Atsumi T., Tonosaki K. Smelling lavender and rosemary increases free radical scavenging activity and decreases cortisol level in saliva. Psychiatry Res. 2007; 150(1): 89-96.

Cavanagh H.M.A., Wilkinson J.M. Biological activities of lavender essential oil, Phytotherapy Research, vol. 16, no. 4, pp. 301–308, 2002.

Dwyer A.V., Whitten D.L., Hawrelak J.A. Herbal medicines, other than St. John's Wort, in the treatment of depression: a systematic review. Alternative Medicine Review, vol. 16, no. 1, pp. 40–49, 2011.

Goerg KJ, Spilker T. Effect of peppermint oil and caraway oil on gastrointestinal motility in healthy volunteers: a pharmacodynamic study using simultaneous determination of gastric and gall-bladder emptying and orocaecal transit time. Aliment Pharmacol Ther. 2003 Feb; 17(3): 445-51.

Gorji A., Ghadiri M. K. History of headache in medieval Persian medicine, Lancet Neurology, vol. 1, no. 8, pp. 510–515, 2002.

Gorji A. Pharmacological treatment of headache using traditional persian medicine, Trends in Pharmacological Sciences, vol. 24, no. 7, pp. 331–334, 2003.

Hirokawa K., Nishimoto T., Taniguchi T. Effects of lavender aroma on sleep quality in healthy Japanese students. Perceptual & Motor Skills, vol. 114, no. 1, pp. 111–122, 2012.

Hongratanaworakit. Stimulating effect of aromatherapy massage with jasmine oil. Nat Prod Commun. 2010 Jan; 5(1): 157-62.

Jager W., Buchbauer G., Jirovetz L., Fritzer M. Percutaneous absorption of lavender oil from a massage oil. Journal of the Society of Cosmetic Chemists, Vol. 43, Pages 49-54.

Jeena K., Liju V.B., Kuttan R. Antioxidant, anti-inflammatory and antinociceptive activities of essential oil from ginger. Indian J Physiol Pharmacol. 2013 Jan-Mar; 57(1):51-62.

Mollace V., Sacco I., Janda E., Malara C., Ventrice D., Colica C., Visalli V., Muscoli S., Ragusa S., Muscoli C., Rotiroti D., Romeo F. Hypolipemic and hypoglycaemic activity of bergamot polyphenols: from animal models to human studies. Fitoterapia. 2011 Apr; 82(3): 309-16. doi: 10.1016/j.fitote.2010.10.014.

Murase T., Misawa K., Haramizu S., Minegishi Y., Hase T. Nootkatone, a characteristic constituent of grapefruit, stimulates energy metabolism and prevents diet-induced obesity by activating AMPK. Am J Physiol Endocrinol Metab. 2010 Aug; 299(2): E266-75. Doi: 10.1152/ajpendo.00774. Epub 2010 May 25.

Nitsa Mirsky (2012). Glucose tolerance factor – Insulin Mimetic and potentiating agent – A source for a novel anti-diabetic medication. Available at: http://dx.doi.org/10.5772/54350.

Perry R., Terry R., Watson L.K., Ernst E. Is lavender an anxiolytic drug? A systematic review of randomised clinical trials. Phytomedicine, vol. 19, pp. 825–835, 2012.

Ranasinghe P., Pigera S., Premakumara G.A., Galappaththy P., Constantine G.R., Katulanda P. Medicinal properties of 'true' cinnamon (*Cinnamomum zeylanicum*): a systematic review. BMC Complement Altern Med. 2013; 13:275.

Shen J., Niijima A., Tanida M., Horii Y., Maeda K., Nagai K. Olfactory stimulation with scent of grapefruit oil affects autonomic nerves, lipolysis and appetite in rats. Neuroscience Letters, Vol. 380, Issue 3, 3 June 2005, Pages 289-294. Epub 2005 Feb 5.

Sigh G., Maurya S., deLampasona M.P. A comparison of chemical, antioxidant and antimicrobial studies of Cinnamon leaf and bark volatile oils, oleoresins and their constituents. Food and Chemical Toxicology, 2007; 45(9): 1650-1661.

Saravanan G. Ponmurugan P., Deepa M.A., Senthilkumar B. Anti-obesity action of gingerol: effect on lipid profile, insulin, leptin, amylase and lipase in male obese rats induced by a high-fat diet. J Sci Food Agric. 2014 Nov;

94(14): 2972-7. doi: 10.1002/jsfa.6642. Epub 2014 Apr 7.

Watanabe E., Kuchta K., Kimura M., Rauwald H.W., Kamei T., Imanishi J. Effects of bergamot (Citrus bergamia (Risso) Wright & Arn.) essential oil aromatherapy on mood states, parasympathetic nervous system activity, and salivary cortisol levels in 41 healthy females. Forsch Komplementmed. 2015; 22(1):43-9. doi: 10.1159/000380989. Epub 2015 Feb 19.

Milton Keynes UK
Ingram Content Group UK Ltd.
UKHW012333010424
440439UK00004B/206